Reality Therapy—A Workable Approach for Adolescents

Reality Therapy—A Workable Approach for Adolescents

Rev. Dr. Shirley McCoy Watson

Edited By: Phenessa A. Gray
Author of My Soul's Surrender

iUniverse, Inc.
New York Lincoln Shanghai

Reality Therapy—A Workable Approach for Adolescents

iUniverse books may be ordered through booksellers or by contacting:

iUniverse
2021 Pine Lake Road, Suite 100
Lincoln, NE 68512
www.iuniverse.com
1-800-Authors (1-800-288-4677)

ISBN-13: 978-0-595-35114-5 (pbk)
ISBN-13: 978-0-595-79816-2 (ebk)
ISBN-10: 0-595-35114-X (pbk)
ISBN-10: 0-595-79816-0 (ebk)

Printed in the United States of America

Contents

Acknowledgement

I am so grateful to my family for supporting me while I was writing this book. My sister, Carlond W. Gray, author of "40 Days: A Personal Journal to Renewal of Mind and Spirit and my neice, Phenessa A. Gray, author of "My Soul's Surrender." The time spent by both of them reviewing the book is appreciated.

Adolescents as well as their parents need as much information as possible to help them through the period from the age of thirteen to twenty-one. Helping parents with tips on how to deal with their children is my focus. Also, sharing information with counselors who read this book with methods to use in counseling as it relates to reality therapy.

Thanks to my friends Dr. Delores Sconias, Lorraine Alston, Jeanetta Lawrence, Julia M. Lamons (my oldest sister), Barbara Gerald, Rev. Kernetta Carter, Dr. Myles Monroe and others who gave me an encouraging word to maximize my potential.

1

Introduction

The purpose of this book is to illustrate how unrealistically adolescents, including boys and girls, view life and the methods thy chose to cope. Often the approach that is used by girls and boys to cope tends to lend itself to futile pursuits-promiscuity, illicit drug and alcohol use, seeking relationships with no promise of a future, etc. I desire to illustrate how reality therapy may be used as a means 1) to help them face reality and reject irresponsible behavior and 2) to develop a positive outlook of the future even though the portrait that has been painted by society appears to be futile.

It is my contention that adolescents have a tendency to look at life (the real world) unrealistically. The realization that life is not characterized by "fun" and "games" but responsibility, moral and ethical values, and good judgment appears to escape many youth today.

For the purpose of this book, the term adolescent will be used to describe teenagers, young people, young adults, and youth. The word "adolescent" means the period of growth to maturity-thirteen to twenty-one years of age. We must realize that adolescence is in an ill-defined period of life which begins prior to the teenage years and extends into the late teens or early twenties. During this time the young person changes physically, sexually, emotionally, intellectually and socially (their personal world). He or she moves away from dependence and the protective confines of the family and toward relative independence and social productivity. The changes sometimes come quickly and immature young people do not always adjust efficiently. This has led some people to conclude that adolescence is a highly disruptive period characterized by rebellion and perpetual turmoil.

Adolescents must realize that they have choices in every situation and that they must be willing to accept the concomitant consequences of each choice. Many youth find themselves involved with the court system at an early age. Status offenders, as defined by the Juvenile Justice Department, are those children who are truants, runaways, and ungovernable. Dependents are those who are dependent upon the state in which they live for their basic needs-food, clothing, and shelter. Delinquents are those who have committed a crime irregardless of the nature or severity of the offense.

Reality therapy is defined in this book as a process in which people are taught better ways to fulfill their needs than they have learned so far. It can relate to girls and boys by teaching them 1) how to avoid and recognize destructive behavior, 2) how to develop healthy respect for themselves and others, 3) ways to build self-esteem and self-worth, 4) provide a healthy and positive perspective about life, and 5) to practice discipline and self-control. When coupled with acceptance and recognition of Jesus Christ as Lord and Savior, they will find themselves enjoying the abundant life which only knowing Christ provides.

Reality therapy focuses on bringing about an understanding of the responsibilities of life. It points out the crisis periods that are experienced due to problems created by one's environment and inner-struggles. It also helps individuals to understand adverse situations that happen in the lives of those close to them-parents, friends. Adolescents experience a significant period of change characterized first by a need to adjust to physical changes, second by the influence of great social pressures, and third by the challenge of making life-determining decisions about values, beliefs, identity, careers, and one's relationship with others, including those of the opposite sex. An adolescent's environment plays a vital part in how he or she relates to society. Many of them see situations handled by others with deceit and trickery. The role modeled by adults appears to be a way of life. This occurs in an effort to hide from or evade the real issues of life. As a result of poor decisions made by many parents, adolescents have a distorted view of how good decision-making skills can influence their position in life.

Adolescents become confused because of the misplaced values of society and the double standard that is also prevalent. While smoking pot is illegal and therefore, by implication, immoral, drinking alcohol is legal and supposedly moral. They find themselves with low self-steem, low self-worth, attitudes of thoughtlessness, manipulative behavior, self-centeredness, and experiencing moral indifference. They find themselves confronted with inherent choices: either accept the values of society or make society accept theirs. They learn that the only standard by which we are judged is by what we do-our action, not our thoughts.

A practical approach to implementing reality therapy in any programmatic setting will be discussed and systematically developed in this analysis. Generalities are not acceptable to young people in today's society. Specific ways of coping are looked for and, if not available, peer pressure prevails-what is accepted by their peers become the norm.

The factors that need to be stressed in reality therapy are "trust" and "friendship." Adolecents must come to realize also that there is no perfect human relationship. The art of "negotiation" and "compromise" is the tool used in learning how to get along with others.

2

Rebellious Youth-Why?

With the awareness that they are no longer children, adolescents seek freedom. They want it in large doses, but handle it better in small and ever-increasing amounts. Often what the young people want and think they can handle differs from what parents are willing or think it wise to give. This can create considerable tension, frustration, power struggles and even rebellion.

Rebellion is merely behavior that denotes defiance of authority or resistance against any power or restriction. Those in resistance against any power or restriction. Those in authority tend to pose a threat to a young person's freedom to express himself or herself. The meaning of freedom in the minds of young adults is the right to express himself or herself in whatever manner they choose without prohibitions. Often this poses a problem because no thought is given with regard to respecting the rights of those around them.

U. S. New and World Report (April 27, 1970) interviewed Dr. William Glasser with regard to rebellious youth. In the interview he said, "what accounts for the alarming rise in violence, use of narcotics and other troubles in schools is a failure crisis. These young people are failing in important areas of their lives. They are doing what they think is best for them at a particular time by running away from reality. They believe they are failures. It is not very useful simply to them immoral."

He further states, "youth are failures in the most important things. classroom achievement, making friends, having fun, winning the respect of others in responsible ways. Successfully children generally don't get into serious trouble. It is when a child starts thinking of himself or herself as a failure and therefore not worth very much that he or she begins to choose to act irresponsible, to strike back at others, including parents."

In my opinion this feeling of failure is more common among young girls today. The proportion of juvenile delinquent girls getting arrested is on the rise. There are indications that more girls are using drugs than in the past and that they are using drugs at lower age levels.

For example, the runaway girl who winds up in a commune in a big city is quite likely to be a failure. She is the withdrawal kid, running away from a reality she can not tolerate. A girl can escape reality by getting involved in illicit sex. She gains confirmation of her role as a woman if she can get someone to have sex with her. She is looking for love in all the wrong places. She does not know the difference in making love (a meaningful relationship between two married people) and sex, merely a lustful act. If she gets pregnant—well, that is still another female role in which she thinks she can be successful.

In the same way, coming under the influence of drugs is an attempt to escape from reality which many young girls who feel failure judge too painful to endure. We have to help them to succeed, to get rid of the pain or we will never reduce narcotics use, the running away, or the promiscuous behavior.

Research has proven that this sense of failure takes hold very early in school life, especially in the central city. Better than nine out of ten delinquents are school failures. For over fifty percent of children school is failure. As a result of these statistis, a great deal of concern is being shown by the educational system in Jacksonville, Florida, Duval County. The City is addressing the needs of adolescents who have been labeled delinquents, habitual drug users and the problems that are encountered by teenage pregnancy. The mayor has formed a task force to address teen pregnancy. Campaigns have been launched by neighborhood community groups (MAD DADS) to address the issue of drugs.

Upon careful review of the issues raised by U. S. New and World Report, I am led to the conclusion that adolescents often rebel not only due to a desire to express themselves, but their sense of failure in life creates an inability to cope with reality. Rebellion is characterized in behavior such as sexual promiscuity, withdrawal, use of narcotics, participation in violent acts, and irresponsibility.

Ways in which reality therapy can counter rebellion are to 1) isolate the problems that are plaguing the youngster, 2) offer an alternative way of coping with the problem to replace the rebellious behavior, 3) get involved and ask questions designed to get the adolescent to evaluate his or her behavior against reality, and 4) help him or her to work out a plan to change his or her behavior and get a commitment that he or she has a reasonable chance of keeping.

The word "adolescent" does not appear anywhere in the Bible. There is a very strong possibility that the biblical writers did not think of adolescence as a separate period of human development. The Bible in Proverbs chapter three speaks on "Guidance for the Young." The Bible does speak on children. It is my belief that instructions given to children would imply that these children were old enough to understand and comply. I would, therefore, assume that biblical teaching on children applied to "children" of adolescent age as well.

The Bible also speaks to "young men" and "young women." In Ecclessiastes chapter eleven verses nine and ten. (LB) the writer says:

> "Young man, it's wonderful to be young! Enjoy every minute of it! Do all you want to; take in everything, but realize that you must account to God for every thing you do. So banish grief and pain, but remember that youth, with a whole life before it, can make serious mistakes!"

The Scripture portrays young people as "visionaries, who are strong, expected to respect their elders, and instructed to humble themselves under the mighty hand of God, that He may exalt them at the proper time, casting all their cares on Him, because He cares for them." We can see in this that considerable guidance is given to young people struggling during adolescence.

I strongly believe that adolescents rebel and are alienated from parents when the parental faith is based on rules, rather than on the Christian virtues of acceptance and forgiveness. Often when the family is concerned more about status, competition and legalism, the young person is more likely to rebel. When parents are inconsistent in their walk with the Lord, young people tend to label them "hypocrites." Adolescents are not interested in legalism and religious talk without corresponding action. They are much more impressed when they can see a "living faith" in their parents lives, characterized by worship, sincere commitment to Jesus Christ, and a daily willingness to serve Him. Adolescents need a firm foundation on which to build lives, formulate values, solve problems and plan for the future. For example, parents who are growing spiritually provide an atmosphere of love, stability, acceptance and forgiveness in the home.

Permission was granted to me by the P. A. C. E CENTER FOR GIRLS to have the students participate in a survey-<u>Rebellious Youth-Why?</u> The purpose of the survey was to gain first-hand information from adolescent girls on this issue. The following statistics provide a breakdown of the participants:

Blacks-7
Whites-25
Spanish American-1

15 years of age-9
16 years of age-12
17 years of age-8
18 years of age-4
Total Surveyed-33

The questions are stated below with the most frequent response quoted.

1. What are some frustration or tension producers young people experience in today's society?

Some frustration or tension producers are a) parental communication and intervention in their lives, b) sex, and c) peer pressure.

2. What are adolescent and/or young adults seeking today?

Adolescents and/or young adults are seeking freedom from parents, independence, money, and self-esteem.

3. Define "FREEDOM" (your words).

Freedom means "not being told what to do by adults;" "being on your own and making your own decisions;" "being able to do what you please;" and "space."

4. How do young people relate to authority figures contacted on a regular basis? (i. e. , teachers, civic leaders, parents)?

Young people relate to authority figures by "just agreeing with them, because they are in control. It is not because you agree with what they do. They have the upper hand." "Even though you agree with them, you build up anger and hostility inside." "Young people do not respect authority and are not afraid of what will happen to them if they rebel."

5. Do you believe in God? Explain.

Thirty-two said, "Yes, I believe in God." One said, "I believe in a higher being but not God." Some of the statements were: "I just do; that is the way I was brought up." "He wakes me up every morning and I serve Him." "I believe but I really don't understand a lot about religion." "Since I was a little girl my mom and grandmother taught me about God and I read my Bible."

6. Do you think young people have a negative outlook on life? If so, why?

Young people have a negative outlook on life, "because of a bitter world." "Some do because they feel like they don't have much to look forward to." "Because they are always talking negative about themselves." "Some kids think everyone is against them."

7. Some young people use rebellion as a tool to survive within their environment. Why?

Some young people use rebellion as a tool, "To get attention." "To keep people from running over them." "To get what they want."

8. STATEMENT: "Most young people who are classified as "troublemakers" are from low-income or deprived families? (What is your opinion)

"Not all bad people are poor." "Anybody can be a troublemaker, even rich people." "I agree, because I think they have been deprived for so long, and from so many things, they have anger built up inside them."

9. Why do young people rebel against authority or rules?

"We don't like being told what to do." "To be a hot-shot, cool, a show-off or to get attention." "To get even with authority."

10. Is negative behavior expressed by young adults directly related to their sense of failure in life? Why?

"Especially if they think they are a loser." "Yes, they decide that they can't live up to others expectations, so they stop trying." "Yes, most young adults are yelled at for mistakes, but not too much is said about how good they are doing."

11. Why do you think young people drop out of school?

"Because they usually get caught up with the wrong crowd or they feel like nobody cares whether they are there or not. You kinda get lost in the shuffel." "They get fed up with the system." "Too many rules. They treat most kids like they are stupid. Some teachers try their best to downgrade students. Others just push them too far."

The information provided by these young people appears to be honest and above board. They were not coached or pressured to answer the questions in any special way.

3

Duval County School Dropout and Teenage Pregnancy Statistics

Statistics from the Duval County School Board reveals the dropout rate for 2003-2004 as follows:

Dropouts By School

School No.	School Name	2003		2004	
		Num	Rate	Num	Rate
33	Robert E. Lee		6.7%	105	6.3%
35	Andrew Jackson		6.2%	63	1.9%
38	Baldwin		0.5%	10	3.0%
75	Paxon		0.8%	11	0.7%
86	Terry Parker		6.6%	125	7.6%
90	Englewood		4.8%	98	11.6%
96	Jean Ribault		5.3%	76	2.9%
107	Douglas Anderson		0.1%	2	0.6%
153	Stanton		0.1%	.	.
165	William M. Raines		4.1%	64	3.2%
223	Duncan U. Fletcher		3.2%	82	4.6%
224	Samuel Wolfson		3.4%	70	5.7%
237	Sandalwood		5.9%	130	3.4%
241	Nathan B. Forrest		7.4%	111	8.0%
248	Ed White		7.4%	147	9.2%
260	Mandarin		1.6%	49	2.2%
265	First Coast		4.8%	89	6.3%
280	Frank H. Peterson		5.8%	40	6.7%
285	A. Philip Randolph		6.0%	52	7.1%
District			4.6%	1324	5.1%
State			3.1%		2.9%

DUVAL COUNTY TEEN BIRTH DATA as of SPRING 2003
The numbers in RED have been updated for 2003

What is the total number of girls (10-19) in Duval County?

		2003
10 to 14	29,097	29,333
15 to 19	27,509	28,789
Total	56,606	58,122

Population Numbers of Ages 10-19 in the following Zip Codes					
	Ages 10-14		Ages 15-19		Totals ages
Zip Codes	Male	Female	Male	Female	10-19
32202	54	83	230	76	443
32204	192	183	185	141	701
32205	1049	941	842	854	3,686
32206	938	927	895	950	3,710
32208	1497	1431	1535	1418	5,881
32209	1782	1882	1622	1495	6,781
32211	1286	1214	1083	1101	4,684
32250	655	648	675	653	2,631
32254	843	767	764	742	3,116
Total	8,296	8,076	7,831	7,430	31,633

Number of Teen Births & Teen Birth Rates by Zip Codes							
Ages 15-19							
Total Zips	2000 TBR	2001 TBR	2000 Counts	2001 Counts	Total Zips	2003 TBR	2003 Counts
32202					32202	DSU	<5
32204	108.37	111.38	22	23	32204	DSU	16
32205	80.05	87.46	69	76	32205	79.63	68
32206	130.53	112.51	121	107	32206	83.16	79
32207	67.88	67.27	71	71	32207	47.23	48
32208	78.22	66.06	111	94	32208	67.70	98
32209	125.00	138.02	189	208	32209	123.75	185
32210	74.58	69.08	152	142	32210	66.44	136
32211	74.33	75.65	86	89	32211	74.48	82
32216	50.97	57.55	50	57	32216	45.55	42
32217	52.16	52.90	35	36	32217	40.66	27
32218	62.16	68.51	91	103	32218	59.01	94
32219	100.00	76.70	35	27	32219	72.83	26
32220	58.54	38.69	24	16	32220	66.19	28
32221	51.95	58.11	36	41	32221	35.63	29
32224	15.82	19.25	20	25	32222	DSU	9
32225	28.33	22.79	43	36	32223	DSU	11
32233	74.38	64.03	63	55	32224	18.39	21
32234	DSU	81.18	<5	22	32225	33.84	58
32244	56.05	57.34	94	98	32226	DSU	11
32246	48.44	43.48	56	52	32233	52.69	51
32250	46.38	37.28	32	26	32234	DSU	15
32254	78.87	93.36	53	64	32244	46.16	89
32256	37.09	36.85	24	25	32246	58.63	71
32257	31.01	24.60	37	30	32250	38.28	25
32277	42.59	38.31	48	44	32254	83.56	62
					32256	42.27	29
					32257	18.65	23
					32258	DSU	14
					32266	DSU	<5
					32277	45.92	54

Page 2

How many teens give birth in Duval county a year?

Number of teen births, 2001	Duval County (2000)	FL (2000)	US (2000)
15- to 19-year-olds	1,522	22,763	468,990
10- to 14-year-olds	30	362	8,519
15- to 17-year-olds	468	7,227	157,209

4

A Model Program for Treatment of Adolescent Girls

The P. A. C. E Center for Girl

"WHY THE NEED?

It has been observed that the experiences of young adolescent females caught up in the Juvenile Justice System were given little attention. The majority of females in trouble with the law was charged with status offenses of which sexually related offences and ungovernable behavior have featured most prominently. The system's reactions to these girls have been to protect them from their environment for their own good. Similar attitudes and standards have not been applied to boys facing charges.

This differential treatment has led to a nationwide absence of resources which would enhance a girl's self-worth, foster independence, and a responsibility for her own destiny and that of her own community. Even though support treatment programs for the delinquent children were in place, it was often easier to have the courts adjudicate this status offender female delinquent for her acts of truancy, incorrigibility, running away and ignore the underlying reasons for her behavior. A lack of women role models employed in the Juvenile Justice System has also contributed to limiting the adolescent girls' adjustment and rehabilitation. particularly at such a time of crisis in her life.

THE PILOT

It started with a dream shared by three women who wanted teenage girls in the Juvenile Justice System in Jacksonville, Florida to have the same opportunity already offered to boys in the same circumstances. On January 7, 1985 the dream became a reality when P. A. C. E. (Practical and Cultural Education Center for

Girls) opened its doors. The six month pilot program started with eleven girls and two full-time staff with one room in a church. Innovation, creativity and enthusiasm had to substitute for amenities, salaries and funds. The girls painted and decorated the room. P. A. C. E. flourished.

Within six months, P. A. C. E. was on the move. Referrals quickly surpassed available openings. After three months, P. A. C. E. moved to the Florida Community College in downtown Jacksonville, Florida. P. A. C. E. continued to respond to Jacksonville's overwhelming demand for an alternative to lockup for this community's adolescent girls in conflict with the law.

P. AC. E. is a unique program, being the only one of its kind in the state. It was formed to address the special needs of teenage girls only. P. A. C. E. is unique in Florida and research has not revealed a similar project nationwide. It is a non-profit, year-round, nonresidential, comprehensive educational program whose goal is to reduce the high school dropout rate (as defined by the pubic schools) among girls fourteen to seventeen years of age. It targets the needs of girls who are economically and socially disadvantaged. In 1988 the statistics showed twenty-five percent of P. A. C. E. 's population were adjudicated dependent by the courts. Fifty percent were status offenders (i. e. , truants, runaways, ungovernable as defined by Health and Rehabilitative Services (HRS), students, psychologists, psychiatrists) and twenty-five percent had violated the law (i. e. , were adjudicated delinquent by the Juvenile Court). In 1986-1987, seventeen percent of the girls at P. A. C. E. were minority. Over eighty percent were from families receiving federal and/or state aid and forty percent lived in a single parent home. P. A. C. E. during this period nurtured, motivated, educated and inspired a minimum of ninety troubled young women and their families each year to become productive income producing citizens, an asset to their community.

In 1995 Duval County recorded the highest number of female status offenders (truants,runaways,ungovernables) in Florida. In 1986 Duval Court recorded the third highest number of live births to mothers under nineteen years of age in Florida and the fourth highest number of live births to unwed mothers under nineteen years of age. Almost one third of the crime committed in Duval by juveniles was committed by females.

In 2003 there were 36, 374 violent crimes committed by adolescents. In 2004 there were 6, 819 violent crimes committed by adolescents, an increase of 7%.

This report was obtained from the Juvenile Justice Department. I was not able to get the breakdown between boys and girls.

P. A. C. E for girls celebrated 20 years of service on February 24, 2005 with an enrollment of 80 girls. The program has served over 2, 000 girls since its inception. The governor of Florida, Jeb Bush, proclaimed January 7, 2005 "Pace Center for Girls Believing in Girls Day." There are currently 19 locations.

PROGRAM OBJECTIVES

(1) To provide a year-round, non-residential, community based, comprehensive, alternative educational program for a minimum of ninety girls per annum ages fourteen to seventeen years of age.

(2) To provide an accredited comprehensive high school education curriculum leading to a high school diploma with credit accumulation or passing the GED (General Education Development) education.

(3) To provide career development vocational skills in the areas of Computer, Secretarial/Word Processing skills, Budgeting & Money Management, Interviewing Skills, and Career Planning by rotating students through these areas within six months.

(4) To enroll each P. A. C. E. graduate in further education and/or a job, or the military upon graduation.

(5) To maintain a minimum of ninety percent attendance in the P. A. C. E, school.

(6) To ensure at least two High School Diplomas are obtained per month by these high risk students.

(7) To maintain a cost efficient/cost effective program within the budget expenditure of similar youth programs for boys.

(8) To maintain one to eight teacher/student ratio.

(9) To have P. A. C. E. students engage in two to three community service projects per month.

(10) To provide students access to P. A. C. E. Instructors/counselors twenty-four hours. To provide a minimum of one Parent/Guardian conference a

month. To provide ongoing counseling for drugs, teenage pregnancy, sexuality, AIDS and dysfunctional families.

(11) Monitor a graduates progress for three years after graduation with up-to-date records regarding living arrangements, family status, employment records, and educational achievements.

Education is the core of P. A. C. E. and <u>key</u> to bringing the majority of the girls out of the mire of broken homes, poverty and low sef-eteem. Each girl attends the P. A. C. E. school and works individually at her own level under the direction of two teachers in a class of a maximum of ten girls at a time. Courses are geared to meet the needs of the students and prepare them for the real world.

5

A Model Program for Treatment of Adolescent Boys

After reviewing several programs for boys, there were two that provided similar services. In 1927, Miss Emily Griffith-renewed Colorado educator, opened "a home for a boy who needs one" -Number 9 Pearl Street in Denver. Over the years thousands of young men have crossed the threshold of this agency. As the service and educational needs of these children changed, so did the programming of what now is the **Griffith Centers for Children.**

Today not only do they treat emotionally troubled young men in the residential units at Larkpur Campus, the Western Campus in Rifle and the South Campus in Colorado Springs, they now offer Foster Care, Adoption and Family Preservation services through the Chins Up Youth and Family Services in the Pikes Peak Region.

Another innovative program was started in September of 1998 by Donnie Read who opened the Liberty Wilderness Crossroads Camp (LWCC). This was an idea that he had three years prior to its opening. This camp is located on 78 acres in the middle of the Apalachicola National Forest on the sight of a former hunting preserve. The camp sports a 50-foot Alpine Climbing Tower, a saw mill, a dorm and an office building. This camp, designed to hold delinquent boys between the ages of 14 and 18.

The Board of Directors includes some of Liberty County's most involved citizens, and they-alone with Read's brothers-brought together an Action Team to develop specific areas such as security, clinical services, continuous care and vocational education. Dr. Wayne Smith, "a local educator, developed a school-to-work model" which is fundamental to the camp's approach. The model focuses on the individual, and took into consideration vocational interest, academic skills, technical abilities, and possibility for community service. The focus is to develop the "whole person." The Liberty Wilderness Crossroads Camp staff has involved local government, mentors, churches, and civic organizations.

A key component to the program at the camp is "continuous Care." Continuous care involves not only working with the camper (or delinquent), but with his family. The camper stays from six to nine months. The Camp has developed an active animal therapy program and is also implementing music, art, and drama therapy. Animal therapy, the use of animals to develop emotional skills in humans, can promote empathy, discipline, self awareness, and heightened perception. These delinquent boys could be in a facility that drives them deeper into criminality rather than one that tries to pull them out of that downward spiral like the Camp. Changes in individual campers come from the integral and holistic approach of the camp.

6

A Workable Approach to Reality Therapy

Many questions have been posed with regard to what is wrong with those who need psychiatric treatment. Question such as "What is it that psychiatrists attempt to treat? What is wrong with the man in a mental hospital who claims he is Messiah; with the boy in and out of detention centers who has burglarized homes and cars; the woman has who continual psychosomatic symptoms of illnesses; the child who has temper tantrums in school and disrupt the class, the man who must lose a promotion because he is afraid to fly, and the bus driver who suddenly goes berserk with a bus load of people careening on a danger-filled ride?"

Regardless of how she or he expresses their problem, everyone who needs psychiatric treatment suffers from one basic inadequacy: she or he is unable to fulfill their essential needs. The extent to which the symptoms are reflected implies the degree to which the person is unable to fulfill their needs. The behavior patterns of patients requiring psychiatric care indicates that in their unsuccessful effort to fulfill their needs, all patients have a common characteristic: they all deny the reality of the world around them. Some deny the rules of society by breaking the law; others claim their friends are plotting against them, denying the reality of such behavior. Some are afraid of crowded places, close quarters, airplanes, or elevators, yet they freely admit that their fears are unfounded. Millions drink to blot out the inadequacy they feel, but that need not exist if they could learn to be different and far too many choose suicided rather than face the reality that they could solve their problems by more responsible behavior. Whether it is a partial denial or the total blotting out of all reality of the chronic backward patient in the state hospital, the denial of some or all of reality is common to all patients. Success in therapy will become a reality when they are able to give up denying the

18

world and recognize that reality not only exists but that they must fulfill their needs within its framework.

A girl who lives in a world of her own and a delinquent girl who repeatedly breaks the law are common examples of two conditions. One, denying the real world and two, trying to fulfill her needs as if some areas of the world did not exist or in defiance of her existence.

The way young girls lead their lives can be improved considerably when reality therapy is applied in a creative and tenacious manner. It is understood that some people are more difficult to treat than others. Regardless of the individual's problem or maturation, with skill, reality therapy could be used successfully with anyone needing help.

Using reality therapy as a workable approach causes us to look at the theory that implies all of us are born with at least two built-in psychological needs: 1) the need to belong and be loved and 2) the need for gaining self-worth and recognition. We spend our lives trying to satisfy these needs, and whenever we can't satisfy them, we suffer. Adolescents acting out unacceptable behavior-indulgence in drugs, truancy, promiscuity-are briefly satisfying their need to be recognized and to feel worthwhile. A depressed person uses depression to ask for help. An alcoholic uses alcohol to feel good and thus gain the false impression that his/her needs are met, even though his/her life is falling apart. This destructive behavior creates problems in relationships with people they need. To help people, therefore, we must help them gain the strength to do worthwhile things with their lives and at the same time become warmly involved with the people they need.

The process of reality therapy is:

Step One: Make friends-Establish a warm, supportive relationship, and insist that clients take a look at the lives they are choosing to lead.

Step Two: Focus upon daily activities and ask what they are doing now. Have the clients choose at least one component of their behavior. Try to select the component of their behavior that they are most likely to admit is their choice to work on.

Step Three: Ask the question: Is what you are doing helping you? Once the person accepts that he or she has chosen any part of his or her behavior, that person is ready for this question. "Is it working out? :" or "Is it what you want to do?" or "Is it the kind of thing that's going to make life better for you in the future?" The importance of this step is to get the person to judge whether or not what he or she is doing is effective right now.

Step Four: Help the client make a plan to do better. Using reality therapy requires a lot of time used in planning and checking with the client on how the plans are being carried out.

Step Five: Commitment to the plan. The client is able to see that "I'm responsible, not only to myself but to my therapist and others who care for me."

Step Six: No excuses.
And Seven—No nourishment. These two go together. When there is commitment to plan, there is no excuse for not following through. When the client does not follow through, the therapist asks the client, When will you get it done? "When an excuse is accepted it is saying to the client," I accept your inadequacy, I accept your misery, I accept your inability to keep your commitment."

Step Eight: Never give up. To approach a person with the idea that, if things don't work, we're going to give up. Always have as your motto "We have just begun to fight."

Step Nine: Once the relationship has developed a level of trust and friendship, introduce the client to Jesus Christ and present the plan of salvation. Incorporating biblical principles is the area of problem solving.

Appendix A provides two case studies of adolescent girls with different problems. Reality Therapy was used in each to guide them in fulfilling the needs that exist in their lives.

7

The Counselor and Counseling

People have crossed over paths who would like to be counselors, simply because this is seen as a glamorous activity of giving advice and helping people solve their problems. Even though counseling is gratifying, it doesn't take long for any of us to discover that counseling also is emotionally draining, hard work. As we see so many people hurting, the counselor experiences feelings of pain. Counseling involves intensive concentration. The counselor has a tendency to blame himself, try hard, and wonder what went wrong when the people fail to improve. There is a tendency to increase the counseling workload as more and more needy people come for counseling. Many counselors push themselves closer to the limits of their endurance. One of the hazards of counseling is that sometimes the counselee's problems remind us of our own insecurities or conflicts and this can threaten our stability or feelings of self-worth.

I want to counsel delinquent girls because from the age of thirteen, I wanted someone to talk to me and to listen to me. I needed someone to help me understand the emotional changes I was experiencing. Education in this area was limited in the Black family. SURVIVAL was the primary focus of the Black family, not spending the time needed to meet the needs of the children. Often I would approach my mother and ask her questions about sex, boys, and the different changes my physical appearance was taking and she would shy away from me and pretend not to hear my questions. If I persisted she would accuse me of being, what is known in the Black community as, "fast" (meaning too knowledgeable about the facts of life). Now, I know that it was a direct result of her inability to relate to me the information requested. Her mother did not talk to her and she did not know how to talk to her girls,

Why do you want to counsel? It is seemingly difficult to evaluate one's own motives. Perhaps this is especially true when we examine our reasons for counseling. Paul Welton states, "A sincere desire to help people grow is a valid reason for becoming a counselor, but there are other reasons which motivate counselors and which interfere with their counseling effectiveness."

Some of the reasons are:

1. Curiosity-The Need for Information. In describing their problems, counselees selees often give interesting tidbits of information which might not be shared otherwise. When a counselor is curious he or she sometimes forget the counselee, pushes for extra information and often is unable to keep confidences. For these reasons, people prefer to avoid curious helpers.

The delinquent girls I counsel are very knowledgeable of the ways of the world for their ages. They are able to detect genuine concern from a curious attitude. Because of the habits that are developed by them while being exposed to "Street Life", they will not allow themselves to be conned or exploited.

2. The Need for Relationship. The need that everyone has to be close and to have intimate contact with at least two to three other people is valid. For some counselees, the counselor will be the close friend, at least temporarily. But what if counselors have no close friends apart from the counselees? In such cases the counselor's need for a relationship may hinder the helping. From the delinquent girl's standpoint of view, she will take this as an opportunity to not only develop a close relationship, but use it as a weapon to manipulate the counselor. I believe that if the counselor is concentrating on meeting his or her need for a relationship, the counselee will be successful in using this tool.

3. The Need for Power. The authoritarian counselor likes to "straighten out" others, give advice (even when it is not requested), and play the "problem solver" role.

Delinquent girls are famous for developing power struggles. If a counselor is determined to exhibit the need for power, constant conflict will be evident in the counseling relationship. Most delinquent girls that I have counseled rebel against authoritarian figures any way, so if a counselor projects this image, they will continue to rebel and will not receive the proper guidance to correct their negative behavior.

4. The Need to Rescue. The rescuer takes responsibility away from the counselee by demonstrating an attitude which says, "You can't handle this; let me do it for you." This has been called the "do-good, "messiah approach. With rebellious girls it is necessary to instill the fact that they are responsible for their own actions. In order to teach them responsibility, the approach should be role modeling, not doing it for them.

Two reasons for counseling delinquent girls are 1) to act as a responsible role model and 2) to provide support for them in helping them to resolve conflicts in their lives. I would make myself available to these girls 24 hours a day so that they would be assured that someone is available to meet their needs.

There are some counselors who succeed and their counseling methods are very successful. Their pronounced characteristics are identified by a personality which radiates sincerity, understanding, and an ability to confront in a constructive manner. They also are skilled in the application of techniques which help counselees move toward specific therapeutic goals.

When Jesus was teaching some of his followers one day, He stated why he had come to earth: to give us life in abundance and in all its fullness. Earlier, in what now is surely the most famous verse in Scripture, Jesus had told God's purpose in sending the 'Son-'that whosoever believes in Him should not perish but have eternal life. Jesus, therefore, had two goals for individuals: abundant life on earth and eternal life in heaven.

The counselor's ultimate goal, as a follower of Jesus Christ, is to show people how to have an abundant life and to point individuals to the eternal life which is promised to believers. In many instances, I have found that the girls I have counseled do not have a religious upbringing. They must be given the basic teachings of Christ in small doses and they must be encouraged to become a follower of Christ so as to enjoy eternal life.

What makes a good counselor? A good counselor shows a great deal of warmth, genuineness and accurate emphatic understanding. The word warmth implies caring, respecting or possessing a sincere, nonsmothering concern for the counselee-regardless of his or her attitude or actions. Jesus showed this when He met the woman at the well. He respected her and treated her as a person of worth. Genuineness denotes that a counselor is "for real"—an open, sincere person who avoids phoniness. The counselor is not thinking or feeling one thing and saying something different. Empathy is displayed when the counselor considers the client in the following manner: What does a counselee think? How does he or she really feel inside? What are the counselee's values, beliefs, inner conflicts and hurts? The ability to "feel with" the counselee is the meaning of accurate empathic understanding.

Many delinquent girls are lacking love. Therefore, when a counselor presents warmth, genuineness and understanding the girls tend to have this need in their life met. A girl experiencing problems in her life, especially morally, does not need condemning but respect for her personhood. She should be made to understand that this respect does not mean that her activities are condoned, nor are they acceptable.

A good counselor must also have a relative absence of immobilizing conflicts, hang ups, insecurities or personal problems. If these situations exists in the counselor's life, when displayed by the counselee the counselor will take her mind off of the counselee and reflect upon her or his own inadequacies. The effective counselor is interested in people, alert to his or her own feelings and motives, more self-revealing than self-concealing, and knowledgeable in the field of counseling.

With delinquent girls, a counselor who has not adequately dealt with the emotion anger, for instance will tend to be short-fused, sensitive and will often take negative behavior personally. Therefore, if this emotion is present, a counselor need to make every effort to resolve any conflict so that the counselee is not made a part of it.

Love is "incomparably the greatest psychotherapeutic agent…something that professional psychiatry cannot of itself create, nor release". The Bible commands and encourages us to love our neighbor as we do ourselves. The Christian counselor has a greater challenge than the conventional therapist: A basic approach to helping someone with their problem is to show love-asking God to love needy people through us and asking Him to make us more loving. There is also a need to develop therapeutic characteristics and attempts to become proficient in the knowledge and use of basic counseling techniques.

Some of the basic techniques that are used in helping situations are (1) Attending-for example, eye contact, posture (relaxed and leaning toward the counselee), and gestures that are natural but not excessive or distracting; (2) Listening-for example, hearing not only what the counselee says but what he or she is trying say and what is left unsaid, sitting still, avoiding looking away from the counselee as he or she speaks, and realizing that full acceptance of the counselee is possible without condoning or sanctioning attitudes or behavior destructive of the counselee or of others; (3) Responding-verbal responses; (4) Leading-That is the counselor slightly anticipated the counselee's direction of thought and responds in a way that directs the conversation; (5) Reflecting-This is a way of letting counselees know that we are "with them" and can understand their feelings or thinking. "You must…"; (6) Questioning-The best questions are those which require at least a sentence or two from the counselee (e. g. , "Tell me about your marriage.") rather than those that can be answered in one word ("Are you married?); (7) Confrontation which means presenting some ideas to the counselee that he or she might not see otherwise. Counselees can be confronted with sin in their lives, failures, inconsistencies, or self-defeating behavior and they should be encouraged to change their behavior or attitudes. Confrontation done in a loving, gentle, and nonjudgmental manner is most effective.

In counseling delinquent girls it is necessary to assure them that they have your undivided attention. If they determine that you are distracted, not listening and inattentive, they will get the impression that you are not genuinely concerned. Confrontation is important in counseling delinquent girls due to the fact they hold in their feelings and will not make the effort to describe them to anyone.

As a Christian counselor, I take as my example Jesus Christ who is described in Isaiah 9: 6 (KJV) as being the Wonderful Counselor. He is the counselor's counselor—ever available to encourage, direct and give wisdom to human people-helpers. It is my firm belief that a Christian Counselor is merely a skilled and available instrument through whom the Holy Spirit works to change lives.

In Romans 12: 8 (KJV) the gift of exhortation (paraklesis-meaning "coming alongside to help") is given and implies such activities as admonishing, supporting and encouraging others. The Message Bible paraphrases' I Corinthians 12: 12-14 as follows:

> "A body isn't just a single part blown up into something huge. It's all the different-but-similar parts arranged and functioning together. If Foot said I am not elegant like Hand, embellished with rings"; I guess I don't belong to this body, would that make it so? If the Ear said, "I'm not beautiful like Eye, limpid and expressive; I don't deserve a place on the head," would you want to remove it from the body? If the body was all eye, how could it hear? If all ear, how could it smell? As it is, we see that God has carefully placed each part of the body right where he wanted it."

The Bible writers express in several scriptures the importance of wise counsel. Several are quoted below which tend to lend themselves as support.

> Proverbs 11: 14 says, "Where no counsel is, the people fall: but in the multitude of Counselors there is safety." (KJV)

> Proverbs 12: 15 says, "The way of a fool is right in his own eyes, but he that hearkened unto counsel is wise." (KJV)

> Proverbs 15; 22 says, "Without counsel purposes are disappointed: but in the multitude of counselors they are established." (KJV)

> Proverbs 27: 9 says, "Ointment and perfume delight the heart, and a sweetness of a man's friend gives delight by hearty counsel."

8

Ways of Gathering Data

Documentation of data is a vital aspect in counseling. The skill of gathering significant data is an asset to a good counselor. Christian counselors in particular are deeply concerned about information on the individual. It is felt that vital information is needed in order to solve the counselee's problems.

There are two ways a counselor may gather data: 1) overtly-when the problems can be clearly identified, and an approach to resolving the problems may be offered without probing, and (2) covertly-this method is applied when the problem is being hidden or not confessed as such; requires probing to determine the problem. Communication is a vital part in data gathering. A counselee communicates in one of two ways: non-verbally and verbally, i. e. , by what kindergarten teachers call the show and tell methods. Non-verbal behavior includes but are not limited to (1) physical symptoms, (2) frequent body movements, (3) voice, (4) dress, (5) slowness, (6) seductive behavior, (7) location of the counselee, (8) laughter, and (9) late or early. Two kinds of data in counseling that correspond roughly to these two methods may be called core data-data given directly by the counselee and halo data-deals with information gathered in such ways as poor eye contact, poor appearance, and poor poster. Some data are given directly by the counselee, usually by word of mouth. But data also may be gathered by observation. Sometimes the halo data is far more important than the core data. Halo data may be derived only from visual and auditory cues, but also from tactile (e. g. the odor of alcohol) cues.

Perhaps the counselees before the counselor are a mother and father who have come, they say, in order to find a way to make their relationships with their delinquent son or daughter more vital. If the counselor listens only to what they say, he or she may find little to go on. So far they may have presented their problem euphemistically; actually, things between the family members are very bad but they are embarrassed to say so. To listen to what the parents say to the child, the counselor might conclude that the parents are model, supportive parents. But when the parents make positive statements about the daughter, the counselor catches the sickening sweet caustic note in their voices, he or she knows that the parents have betrayed resentment and anger because they have been placed in this position. At this point this halo datum is much more important than their words. How words are spoken discloses the true attitude of the speaker.

As observant counselor notes the way that Kim glares at her parents whenever they bring up the question of her friends. "In that area," the counselor tentatively concludes, "I suspect I shall find serious problems." He or she makes the notation "friends" in the agenda column of his or her Weekly Counseling Record, (See Appendex B) and as soon as it is appropriate begins to probe the area. Nor will he or she fail to note that the mother seems to do everything that she can to keep from discussing the child's relationship with her father. Whenever the subject seems to be coming up, she jumps in with both feet and tries to avoid the topic or turns the discussion to a safer subject. The halo data clearly reveals that here is another sore spot. Every counselor must learn to look (feel, taste, smell) and listen for halo data. He or she looks at clothing and appearance. Changes in these may provide positive or negative indications of the direction that counseling is going. He or she watches for signs of embarrassment, nervousnesss, tension, blushing, evasion, redirection of conversation, appearance, clothing, etc. When a counselee is pondering an answer to a question, or when he or she is listening to a third person speak, is the time when Halo data are often most apparent.

Core data relies primarily upon questioning. A counselor must learn how to ask questions and probe into answers that are received in order to elicit the information that is needed to understand the problems and be able to help the counselee. Core data gathering is said to be more substantive and more specific than halo data.

For example, a counselor may say something like this when the process of gathering data begins: "We must work out a plan from the Scriptures that will help you to solve your problem (s) in God's way. But first, I will need detailed, accurate data to work with. As we lay out the data, we can lay out a plan."

A Personal Data Inventory (Appendix C) is important when a plan of action is being developed. The answers to the following questions will provide enough information to begin treatment: (1) What is your problem? ; (2) What have you done about it? ; (3) What can we do? ; (4) As you see yourself, what kind of person are you? Describe yourself; (5) What, if anything, do you fear? ; and (6) Is there any other information we should know? .

If organic illness is at the root of the matter the counselor will discover the source of the problems by asking further questions. Whatever appears to be the problem, it is up to the counselor to probe and acquire the necessary information to determine a suitable treatment plan.

Most teenage girls have a tendency to paint a picture laced with emotions, lack of hope, and sheer desperation. They feel that their problems are unsolvable and that their parents are not providing any answers. The answer to the question, "What could be done?", is that the counselor must impress upon the minds of these teenagers that God has the answer; that there is a solution to every problem; and that all they need to do is to <u>find</u> it and <u>do</u> as God says.

One method of focusing in on a problem is to ask the question, "What do you really believe is causing your problem?". If no answer is given, make it a homework assignment. Then ask the counselee to write down how they feel about the problem. Whatever the content of their answers, the counselor is able to develop an approach to dealing with the problem (s) described.

9

Reality Therapy and Drug Abuse

Drug addiction is not a problem that is new. History has recorded over and over again that a certain percentage of people have had serious trouble with drugs whenever or wherever they have been used. Heroin and cocaine, two hard drugs, were problems in western societies. In some cultures, opium or marijuana have been the problem drugs.

The most common thing that is recognized in those who are addicted to a drug is that they change moods. In keeping with this, drugs can be placed on a scale ranging from those with highest potential for addiction to those with lowest potential. "The scale shows the highest potential as heroin, morphine, Demerol, cocaine, barbiturates, amphetamines and alcohol. The lowest potential drugs are tranquilizers-minor "sleeping pills", codeine, bromids, nicotine, marijuana, and caffeine."

Psychological and physical dependency on the above drugs occurs when a person is exposed to a high dosage for a long enough period of time. For example, with heroin the length of time to become addicted need not be long and the effects are both fast and very dangerous; with caffeine the time is longer and the effects are almost unnoticeable.

An individual is said to be addicted when a chemical interferes with the productivity, tranquility, efficiency or well-being of his or her family life, social life, vocational life, and spiritual life. Physical addiction is evidenced when an effort is made to withdraw and the individual becomes physically ill.

In my work with adolescent girls, it is my impression that teenagers consider illicit drugs one of life's commonplaces. This attitude has been developed through their friends and their families, in the magazines they read, the movies they watch, at parties, at home and in school.

According to a report published by the Correctional Officers Association of Florida, Inc. ," A survey of more than 1, 000 high school students in New York City and its suburbs, and dozens of interviews with parents, drug counselors and teenagers themselves conducted by the <u>New York Times</u> clearly indicate that today's young people are more immersed in the drug culture than any before them have been, and at a far younger age.

In talking with some of the adolescent girls at the Practical and Cultural Education Center for Girls (P. A. C. E), it was evident that the message conveyed was even if they have never smoked marijuana, taken pills that were not prescribed for them or used cocaine themselves, most young people know someone who has. Drug use is all around them, from the men who proffer (present for acceptance) marijuana cigarettes in midtown Jacksonville to the neighborhood parks where marijuana smoke is ripe on the breeze, from the adult who takes tranquilizers to cope with daily stress to the movies in which the punch line is cocaine or quaaludes.

Many of the adolescent girls felt that using drugs was making it a rite of passage for them to either be a part of the crowd or not an outsider. Most of these girls do not have a religious background and lack the knowledge of Scripture that teaches the beautiful relationship that someone may have with Jesus Christ in their life. Them "wanting-to-be-a-part-of-the-crowd symdrome" merely comes from lack of acceptance of self, self-worth, and low-self esteem. These girls must be made to realize that Jesus Christ made it possible for us to become children of a heavenly Father who accepts us just as we are. He also considers us as "joint-heirs" with Jesus Christ (we are considered sons an daughters of God the Father). This knowledge provides the basis for having self-worth and a consciousness of being important.

A sixteen year old who smokes marijuana today has no difficulty feeling a little guilty about using it and almost no fear of being arrested. The sixteen year old who does not smoke often feel substantial peer pressure to join in. Some parents may not mind and even look the other way. One of the main reasons for this attitude is that a significant number of parents smoke marijuana and an even greater number drink alcohol.

Naomi Barber, who is the director of a counseling program in a Bronx School District, was quoted as saying, "There's a very different atmosphere to work in today. Ten years ago if a kid even mentioned marijuana, his parents wanted to send him or her to reform school, you knew he or she was a drug addict, he or she was breaking the law. , That was no good. But today a lot of adults think it is perfectly all right. The attitude that it is no worse than a drink of alcohol."

One of the adolescent girls that I interviewed at the Pace Center for Girls stated the following. "There are two groups of children in my school, the jocks and the burn-outs. The burn-outs smoke and take pills and drink, and the jocks are really into sports. You either take one way or the other. If you are not good at sports, you don't have that much of a choice. "At this point, I asked her if she was aware that there is another choice and that being to accept Jesus Christ as Lord and Savior. She replied, "Kids really are not in to religion."

The answer to the question "Why do children use drugs?" can be safely said to be the crisis experienced by adolescents trying to find their identity, availability, and acceptability. They also feel lonely, inadequate, and are unhappy.

It is my opinion that focusing on drugs is not the answer. Focus should be placed on character and helping adolescents to cope with becoming mature adults. They also should be introduced to Jesus Christ and given guidance using principles outlined in Scripture. Even though the Bible does not speak directly to the problem of drugs, it does speak to the use of wine in Proverbs chapter twenty-three verses twenty-nine and thirty and Proverbs chapter thirty-one verses four through seven. It is wrong to buy, sell, condone, possess, or use any drugs illegally. The Bible instructs us to obey the law of the land (Romans chapter thirteen).

Effective counseling is a direct result of showing concern and empathy for the addict. The addict does not need to be criticized, coaxed, pushed to make a promise to stop, threatened, preached at, and ladened with guilt.

Reality therapy in drug addiction seeks to 1) get the individual to acknowledge that there is a problem, 2) provide support, and 3) encourage self-understanding and a change of lifestyle (to include Jesus Christ).

The home is the place where the prevention begins. When a child is respected, loved, disciplined and raised by sensitive, concerned, stable parents, there is greater opportunity for healthy maturing and less likelihood of chemical dependence. A greater sense of security and self-esteem, accompanied by a greater ability to handle the problems of life without drugs exists when a child's emotional needs are met in the home, when they are helped to cope with stress, and when they are taught a clear set of values.

Other considerations that may be a factor in preventing a child from becoming addicted to drugs are 1) instilling a healthy religious faith, 2) providing education on drugs, 3) teaching them how to cope with life, and 4) providing realistic adult examples.

A survey of high school students use of drugs indicates the following: To the question, "Have you ever used drugs?", the results were: Marijuana (54) said "Yes" and (46) said, "No"; Cocaine (15.2) said, "Yes" and (84.8) said, "No"; Pills (not prescribed for respondent) (19.6) said, "Yes" and (80.4) said, "No"; PCP (commonly know as Angel Dust) (93.7) said, "Yes" and (96.3) said, "No"; Quaalude (71.8) said, "Yes" and (92.2) said, "No"; and Heroin (06.6) said, "Yes" and (99.4) said, "No." This information was provided by the Correctional Officers Association.

10

Ways of Using Homework

Homework can be used as an effective tool in good counseling. A counselor who perfects his or her ability to give homework will soon notice the difference in his or her effectiveness in helping people. Making the counselee a part of problem-solving gives him or her a feeling of being included. When a counselor learns how to give good homework assignments, homework that is biblical, homework that is concrete, and homework that creatively fit's the situation, the results will prove that it was worth the time and effort.

One way of using homework is the use of the conference table. Encouraging clients to set up a conference table helps them to use a practical method of achieving the goals set forth in Ephesians 4. Choosing a table that is not used for other purposes, families are asked to sit down each evening and confer about their problems. A table is important for several reasons. Tables tend to bring people together. Writing can be done easily at a table. The time it takes to set up the table may be important for cooling tempers (Proverbs 15: 28; 14: 17), and it is harder to walk away from a discussion when the parties are seated. The table will become a place where previous problems have been solved and a sign of hope.

When parents experience adolescents having problems that are not being addressed in a constructive manner, the conference table can serve as a tool to create an atmosphere that says to the child she or he is being heard. The opportunity is presented for the child to express his or her feelings and to indicate whether he or she feels has a workable solution. In my experience working with delinquent girls, the all-too-frequent comment made by them is, "My parents don't have the time to listen to me." A conference table setting causes each participant to channel their attention and focus their attention on the situation at hand.

Experience in counseling has shown that very few persons who come for counseling have been in the habit of solving interpersonal problems daily. This is to some extent the reason why they are having difficulty. It is apparent that people who have been nursing grudges and building up resentments for a long time find concrete structure helpful in changing old patterns and establishing new ones. One of the most realistic ways of resolving difficulties that have arisen is setting aside a definite period of time towards the end of the day for the family members to meet together and talk over the day's problems.

In order to be effective, the rules for the conference table must be kept simple. In keeping with God's order of the family, the father calls the meeting and is usually in charge. The mother records anything that needs to be put in writing. Prayer should be offered before and after the meeting. In an effort to apply God's principles, the Bible is used during the conference to discover God's will concerning the questions before the family members. The inclusion of the Bible as a tool in resolving problems is dependent upon the counselor having effectively emphasized the need for a Christ-centered conference and having caused the family to come to a saving knowledge of Jesus Christ (both as Savior and Lord).

Models are another way of solving other problems through homework. One of the best ways to learn to put on God's ways is to observe those who have already learned to do them. In my opinion, modeling is an essential biblical method for teaching. Adolescents are accustomed to observing others and making decisions based upon their appeal to pattern their lives by what they see and admire.

Paul teaches in II Thessalonians Chapter three about discipline. This Scripture indicates that there were Christians in Thessalonica who, because they had heard (wrongly) that the second coming of Christ was imminent, thought they could abandon their work. They then went about as busybodies, eating and sponging off others. Their conduct was called "unruly" (or, literally, "undisciplined"). Paul admonished the people, in the name of our Lord Jesus Christ, that ye keep aloof (or withdraw) from every brother who leads an unruly life. The word translated "unruly," means a disorderly kind of life, a life without order or arrangement. The ideas of being "out of place, "out of order" are inherent in the world.

Undisciplined adolescents are most likely to be in the company of individuals who are unruly and who are undisciplined. The counselor will need to encourage the adolescents to find wholesome company to be a part of in order to redirect their lives and behavior in a positive fashion. Individuals who display good moral judgment, virtuous behavior and positive attitudes should be found. The need to learn how to structure their lives is important. Paul directed his readers in the fourth chapter of Philippians not only to pray and concentrate upon the things that were honorable, right, pure, lovely, and of good report, but he continued: "The things you have learned and received and heard and seen in me, practice these things: and the God of peace shall be with you." (Philippians chapter four verse nine) (LB). In Philippians Chapter three verse seventeen, Paul writes, "Brethren join in following my example, and observe those who walk according to the pattern that you have seen in us. (LB).

If an adolescent child has low self-esteem and has a tendency to emphasize the negative things in life, a good homework assignment would be to have him or her look for the positive things that happen in his or her life and to write them down. During the day, she or he should be encouraged to observe the positive things in the life of someone she or he admires and imitate them. When he or she catches him or herself saying negative things, immediately find something positive to say.

Adolescents who feel that their parents are never right should be encouraged to think about his or her actions before rebelling. Consider the motive behind what the parents are doing and try to understand their love for them. They should also be encouraged to consider the consequences of making an unwise decision-to go against their parents' wishes.

The counselee should be encouraged to keep a journal of activities which would include his or her feelings and the emotions experienced. This journal should be done daily on a consistent basis in order to establish a pattern for specific behavior. By doing this, the counselor is able to develop methods to approach the needs that are evidenced in the information provided.

11

Conclusion

Of all the issues discussed in this book, perhaps the factor that stands out more than any is the fact that a spiritual basis must be established by parents at an early age in order to prevent many of the problems experienced by adolescents. Many parents have a tendency to protect teenagers from the stresses of life, but this is both impossible and poor child-rearing. Instead, we should seek to help young people mature without the painful unnecessary consequences that come when there is a breaking of the law, sexual immorality, severe emotional disturbance, inability to succeed academically, interpersonal conflict, or loss of faith.

In the Old Testament, God's instruction to Adam and Eve was to "be fruitful and multiply, and fill the earth." This divine command was obeyed and the whole world quickly filled with people. A large family in Old Testament times was considered a source of special blessings from God and childlessness was regarded with reproach. The modern trend is to limit the size of the family, but children are still important. In Luke Chapter eighteen verses fifteen through seventeen (KJV), Jesus showed them special attention and He lauded their simplicity and trust.

The Bible quickly points out that children are a gift from God and are able to bring both joy and sorrow. In all of Scripture, God tells us that children are to be loved, honored and respected as persons; they are important to God's kingdom and they are not to be harmed. Psalm One Hundred Twenty-seven verse three (KJV) says: "Lo, children are an inheritance of the Lord: and the fruit of the womb is his reward." Children are also given responsibilities: to honor and respect parents, care for them, listen to them and be obedient, One concise Scripture more than all states this in Ephesians Chapter six verses one through three (KJV). "Children obey your parents in the Lord, for this is right. Honor thy father and thy mother which is the first commandment with a promise; that it may be well with thee, and thou mayest live long on the earth."

Parents have a responsibility to love their children, to model mature Christian behavior, to care for their needs, to teach the children and to discipline fairly. We read in Ephesians chapter six verse four (KJV) "And ye fathers, provoke not your children to wrath: but bring them up in the nurture and admonition of the Lord." Children are to be disciplined, but within the instructions given by the Lord.

There are three methods in rearing children that parents have access to and they are 1) by example, 2) by direct instruction and 3) encouragement. Children are provoked to bitterness and discouragement when they are abused physically, psychological (by humiliating them and failing to treat them with respect), neglect, misunderstood intentionally, given expectations that are too high, not loved unless they perform, forced to accept goals or ideas, and when we refuse to admit our mistakes in raising children. Severe emotional disturbances occur when children are sexually abused by parents.

Children thrive on being accepted by parents. In many instances parents will use this as a weapon to force the child to exceed academically. Often this creates a stressful atmosphere for the child. This occurs especially if the child has a problem grasping and simulating the information presented by the teacher. The child becomes more and more confused. If the parents are raising their children according to the Scripture, their love will be unconditional.

Reality therapy clearly emphasizes that it is not easy to be an adolescent or to help young people through their adolescent years. Young people reach adulthood often in remarkable shape, even with the traumatic changes that occur and the adjustments required in their lives.

Adolescents need parents to help bring about an understanding of the responsibilities of life. However, I have noticed that the need for direction in the lives of adolescent girls is more apparent. The main focus of parents is to help them to understand their inner struggles and provide positive ways for them to deal with their environment. Adolescent girls have a need to be educated about the physical changes that occur in their bodies; thereby being made aware of the consequences of illicit sex and promiscuity.

An adolescent's environment plays a significant role in how he or she relates to it. I believe that more attention should be given to the adjustments that are to be made by adolescents due to the fact that their reputation, if scarred, most often is irreparable. Society has a tendency to stress the image of a female more so than that of a male. A young male is expected to make mistakes. In the eyes of society he is just "soaring his oaks." The female is different in that her role is already defined-wife, mother, supporter and help meet.

Jesus told his followers that they had one basic responsibility to complete in His absence: to make disciples. Parents are as disciples. Their primary responsibility is to bring up their children in the fear and admonition of God. They are to prepare them to be disciples using the principles of the Word of God that have been instilled within them. Included in disciplining is teaching them 1) how to avoid and recognize destructive behavior, 2) how to develop a healthy respect for themselves and others, 3) ways to build self-esteem and self-worth, 4) how to provide a healthy and positive perspective about life, and5) to practice discipline and self-control.

As children become teenagers, parental discipline should move into parental discipleship, teaching by word and example how to be a follower of Jesus Christ. Teenagers are "too big to spank," but they are old enough to respond to persuasion, fairness, logic, interest, positive reinforcement, love, parental example, and the power of prayer. Counselors and parents are to help adolescents to grow into Christian personal maturity.

Rebellion is brought in check when a child is 1) taught how to win the respect of others in responsible ways, 2) made to feel loved, accepted, appreciated, and important, and 3) accepted for who he or she is. Often parents try to live out their lives through their children. For example, the father wanted to become a doctor but was unable to get financial assistance. Now, the father sees an opportunity to influence his son or daughter's life by strongly suggesting that he or she become a doctor.

Adolescents want to see their parents "faith in action." A firm commitment by parents will be noticed and admired. When parents present a firm foundation most adolescents will respond and formulate good values, have a basis to resolve problems and have principles to plan for their future.

Parents are encouraged to look at the following themes that are apparent in problems between parent and child. First, instability in the home. When parents are not getting along with each other, children feel anxious, guilty and angry. Second, parental failures. When children are rejected subtly or overtly, nagged and criticized excessively, punished unrealistically (or not at all), disciplined inconsistently, and shown love spasmodically (if at all), then children often experience personal problems or show disruptive behaviors which in turn are annoying to their parents. Third, unmet needs. Some of the most basic needs of growing children are significance, security, acceptance, love, praise, discipline, and the need for God. Fourth, the neglect of the Spiritual. Psalm seventy-eight verses one through eight (KJV) emphasizes that it is important to teach children about God, remember His faithfulness, and not become unruly, stubborn, or rebellious.

As we look at the girls in the program at the P. A. C. E. Center for Girls, all of the above biblical principles apply. Even though many of these girls were never raised in a Christian home, nor were they exposed to biblical teachings, still a basic love and trust as Jesus taught would have kept each of them out of much of the trouble which brought them to this place.

It is the purpose of this writer to instill in each adolescent with whom I come in contact with those biblical principles discussed in this book. Although this counselor can not become a surrogate mother to them, I can be the teacher who shows them, through the methods of reality therapy, how Jesus can make a difference in their lives. If they accept His principles, they can stay out of detention facilities, out of alternative educational programs like this one and out of prison later.

It is the fervent prayer of this writer that she will be used by God's Holy Spirit to plant the seeds of His love and guidance in the life of each adolescent with whom she comes in contact with.

APPENDIX A

CASE #1: PAT

Pat is a fifteen year old female who lives with her mother and father. There are four other children in the home who range in ages for six to thirteen. Pat's mother, who has never worked, is completely illiterate and Pat's father, who is disabled, has not worked for several years. Their monthly income consists of food stamps, Medicaid, and a disability check-all of which keep the family well under the poverty level.

Pat was placed in a seventh grade Child Development Program (CDP) class for chronic truancy, fighting and not participating in class. She was embarrassed by her size (height and weight), as well as her family's financial and educational situation, so the peer pressure just added more to her insecurities. She cannot transfer to another school due to transportation-they do not own a car and it's a three mile walk to the bus stop, not to mention the money it takes to ride. She is really not old enough to work yet, nor are there any places close enough to walk to work.

Recently, Pat was proposed to by a twenty-four year old high school dropout. She is seriously considering the idea. Staying in school is difficult, not to mention that she will not receive a dipolma anyway while in CDP classes. Getting married would get her out of her home-away from the yelling, screaming, fighting and frustration. It would also mean one less person to worry about feeding and clothing, so she could make it a little easier for her parents.

Treatment Plan

To reach Pat, it will take some creativity and flexibility due to what I describe as her sense of doom and failure. She will need to become aware of the fact that her environment-an illiterate mother, disabled father, and the family's financial situation-is a fact of life.

Befriending Pat, winning her confidence and trust will be major factors in her therapy. It is my opinion that adolescents in Pat's situation tend to feel that no one really understands their plight. Most often the only way they see how to resolve their problems is to seek the easiest way out. The first opportunity that knocks usually is received with great anticipation and high expectations.

Pat is embarrassed about her size, height and weight. Often when individuals begin to find things wrong with themselves it is a sign of the onset of a depressed attitude. It takes almost no effort to slip into a pattern of negative thinking-seeing the dark side of life and overlooking the positive. But negative thinking can lead to depression and when the depressed person continues to think negatively, more intense depression results. When Pat is made to realize that in Christ she can be all sufficient, she will develop a positive attitude about life and her problems.

The approach I would take with Pat is to give her optimistic reassuring statements, share ways to overcome depression, ask questions, patiently encourage Pat to talk, and give her periodic compliments. Since Pat is having difficulty in school, she may feel like a failure. She should be made to understand that failure simply means that nobody is perfect, that we have made a mistake and should try to act differently in the future.

She should be encouraged to evaluate her thoughts and attitudes toward life. She will be encouraged to identify her stronger qualities and shown how to set herself up for little successes. She needs to be warned not to set her goals so high that she create an atmosphere of failure.

Biblical principles would be introduced to her gently. Introducing Jesus Christ to her will be important. More importantly will be her acceptance of Him into her life. In introducing her to biblical principles, every effort will be made not to inundate her with religious jargon, rules or legalism. I will help her see that when Christ becomes the center of one's life, there becomes a lot of peace and assurance in the midst of problems. True joy, acceptance and love comes from knowing Jesus and allowing Him to become her "friend." Knowing our position in Christ provides a great deal of confidence and self-worth.

CASE #2: SANDY

Sandy is a pregnant sixteen year old trying to decide whether she should keep her baby or give him or her up for adoption. The father of the baby left town. She lives with her mother who has not worked for many years due to health problems. Their monthly income consists of a small Aid to Families with Dependent Children (AFDC) check and food stamps. Medicare pays medical bills. Sandy's mother wants her to have the baby and give it to her, so that she can continue to receive AFDC checks. When Sandy turns eighteen, the AFDC checks stop.

She and her mother live in a Housing and Urban Development (HUD) facility. She has a history of drug involvement and running away, so in turn has spent time in the detention center. Sandy is presently studying for her General Education Development Examination (GED), but she was enrolled in Child Development Program (CDP) classes while in school. She does not think she can pass the test.

Her education seems to be important to her so she would like to give up her baby so that she can go on with her education or get a job. Often when frustrated, she sees herself like her mother: dependent on welfare, without anything.

Treatment Plan

It is obvious that Sandy is a victim of the "**Independent Syndrome**." I label it as such because many children who are born into or who are in families that are dependent upon the state for support are many times themselves caught up in that "vicious circle." As a result of their dependency upon the state for their basic needs-food, clothing, shelter and medical care-individuals have a tendency to lose the motivation to provide for themselves. It is from observation, the children have a tendency to have a sense of being "trapped" into a lifestyle that is often looked upon as degrading.

Teenage pregnancy has become an alarming concern of educators. Sex Education is being introduced in the educational system in an effort to avoid what Sandy is now having to experience. Often peer pressure is a direct influence on adolescents like Sandy. She should be questioned as to her reasons for becoming sexually active. Two needs appear to have been a direct result of her sexual involvement: the need for acceptance and the need to belong. It is my opinion that she did not focus on the consequences of her actions.

It appears that Sandy, at this point, is probably in a state of confusion, experiencing disappointment and hurt. As a result of the father leaving town, she most likely is experiencing a sense of rejection, feelings of guilt, insecurity, and loneliness. With this in mind, signs of anger, a loss of self-esteem, and anxiety about the future should be looked for.

In providing counseling to her, there will be a need to be sensitive, calm, compassionate and secure enough to tolerate her outbursts of anger. When confronted, the hurt that she is feeling just might be expressed in a negative fashion. Part of that anger most likely will be directed at her mother for wanting to use her situation as an avenue to remain "dependent" upon the state for financial support. Often I have witnessed this as a "tool" by those who feel trapped into the system. This pressure from her mother may cause her to negate her desire to place the child up for adoption. She might be encouraged to look at the option of keeping the baby herself and raising the child by getting help from parenting classes. Even though her mother may not be able to provide for her the better things of life and has placed her in a poverty type setting, she still "loves" her and will try to please her.

Options must be given to her. She must be encouraged to follow her own convictions. She must be given positive reinforcement and encouragement. She should be made aware that she does not have to be "trapped" in the "dependent syndrome." She should be made to feel good about herself and to be shown ways to deal with the guilt she is experiencing. She must realize that her education is important to her future existence. She needs to be educated about such things as dignity and self-worth.

Biblical principles are essential in the lives of young people today. There is no evidence of her having a religious upbringing. The family does not currently appear to be providing a spiritual base. The Bible teaches in Proverbs chapter 3, verses five and six. "Trust in the Lord with all thine heart; and lean not unto thine own understanding. In all thy ways acknowledge Him, and He shall direct thy paths."(KJV)

Sandy will needs to consider addressing the issues in her life by making a commitment to Jesus Christ and afterwards provided biblical principles and scriptures that meet her needs.

APPENDIX B

WEEKLY COUNSELING RECORD

_____
Counselor's Initials

Name_____ Date: _____

Session No. _____

Evaluation of Last Week's Homework   AGENDA

Drift of the Session

APPENDIX C

PERSONAL DATA INVENTORY

IDENTIFICATION DATA:

Name_____ Phone_____

Address_____

_____

Occupation_____

Employer_____ Business Phone_____

Sex_____ Birth Date_____ Age_____ Height _____

Marital Status: Single_____Going Steady_____Married_____

Separated_____ Divorced_____ Widowed _____

Education (last year completed) _____ (grade) Other training
(list type and years) _____

_____

Referred by_____ Relationship _____

HEALTH INFORMATION:

Physical Condition (check one) Very Good _____ Good _____ Average_____

Declining _____ Other_____

Weight _____lbs. Weight changes recently:

Lost _____ Gained _____

List present or past illnesses or injuries or handicaps:

_____

Date of last medical examination _____ Results _____

Your physician's name _____ Address _____

_____

Are you presently taking medication? Yes ___ No ___ If yes, what? _____

_____

Have you used drugs for other than medical purposes? Yes ___ No ___ If so, what?

_____

Have you ever had a severe emotional upset? Yes _____ No _____
Explain_____

_____

Have you ever been arrested? Yes _____ No _____If yes explain.

_____

Will you sign a release of information form so that your counselor may write for social, psychiatric, or medical reports?
Yes _____ No _____

Have you recently suffered the loss of someone who was close to you? Yes _____
No _____ Explain _____

_____

RELIGIOUS BACKGROUND:

Denominational preference: _____ Member _____
Church Attendance per month (circle): 0 1 2 3 4 5 6 7 8 9 10+
Church attended in childhood _____Baptized?
Yes _____ No _____

Religious background of spouse (if married) _____
Do you consider yourself a religious person? Yes _____ No _____
Uncertain _____
Do you believe in God? Yes _____ No _____ Uncertain _____
Do you pray to God? Never _____ Occasionally _____ Often _____

Have you accepted Christ as Lord and Savior of your life? Yes _____
No ____ Not sure what you mean _____
Have much do you read the Bible? Never ____ Occasionally _____ Often ____
Do you have regular family devotion? Yes _____ No _____
Explain   recent   changes   in   your   religious   life,   if   any
_____

_____

TREATMENT HISTORY:

Have you ever had any psychotherapy or counseling before? Yes ____ No ____
If yes, list counselor or therapist and dates:

_____

_____

_____

_____

_____

What was the outcome? _____

Circle any of the following words which best describe you now: active ambitious self-confident persistent nervous hardworking impatient impulsive moody often-blue excitable imaginative calm serious easy-going shy good-natured introvert extrovert likeable leader quiet hard-boiled submissive lonely self-conscious sensitive other

_____

Have you ever felt people were watching you? Yes _____ No _____

Do people's faces ever seem distorted? Yes _____ No _____

Do you have difficulty distinguishing faces? Yes _____ No _____

Do colors ever seem too bright? _____ Too dull _____

Are you sometimes unable to judge distance? Yes _____ No _____

Are you afraid of being in a car? Yes _____ No _____
Is your hearing exceptionally good? Yes _____ No _____
Do you have problems sleeping? Yes_____ No _____

MARRIAGE AND FAMILY INFORMATION

Name of spouse _____ Address _____
_____
Phone _____ Occupation _____
Business Phone _____
Your spouse's age _____ Education (in years) _____
Religion _____

Is spouse willing to come for counseling? Yes _____ No _____
Uncertain _____

Have you ever been separated? Yes _____ No _____
When? _____

Date of marriage _____ Your ages when married: Husband _____
Wife _____

How long did you know your spouse before marriage?
_____
Length of steady dating with spouse _____
Length of Engagement_____

Give brief information about any previous marriages: _____
_____
Information about children:

PM*	Name	Age	Sex	Living Yes No	Education in years	Marital Status

*Check this column if child is by previous marriage.

If you were reared by anyone other than your own parents, briefly explain:

_____

_____

How many older brothers _____ Sisters _____ do you have?

How many younger brothers _____ Sisters _____ do you have?

BRIEFLY ANSWER THE FOLLOWING QUESTIONS:

1. What is your problem?

_____

2. What have you done about it?

_____

3. What can we do? (What are your expectations in coming here?)

_____

4. As you see yourself, what kind of person are you? Describe yourself.

_____

_____

5. What, if anything, do you fear?

_____

_____

6. Is there any other information we should know?

978-0-595-35114-5
0-595-35114-X